HINDSIGHT

Kay J. Tabbert

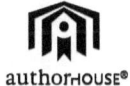

authorHOUSE®

AuthorHouse™
1663 Liberty Drive, Suite 200
Bloomington, IN 47403
www.authorhouse.com
Phone: 1-800-839-8640

First published by AuthorHouse 11/12/2007

ISBN: 978-1-4343-3112-0 (sc)

Printed in the United States of America
Bloomington, Indiana

This book is printed on acid-free paper.

HINDSIGHT

When I was young, if I heard the phrase "hindsight is 20/20," I never gave it a second thought. But, as I got older, I thought it probably meant, "If I only knew then, what I know now." But now that I'm in my 60's and retired, that phrase has taken on a whole new meaning. It seems there is so much I didn't know back then, but rather than wanting to change what has taken place in the past or do it over again, I instead have a growing appreciation for all that's gone before in my life.

On a recent trip to antique stores looking for vintage buttons and lace, I found myself surrounded by so many familiar items from my childhood, that it took me back to the time in my life when every day was filled with surprises and laughter. I've also noticed that the older I get, the more I reminisce about my past, and the more I remember people and events from years ago. Looking back, things from long ago seem so very clear, almost as if it was just yesterday.

MOM AND DAD...BEFORE THE KIDS

Mom and Dad (Emma and Lester Gaertner) "eloped" on January 19, 1934. I've heard they drove for hours that morning in the freezing rain to Angola, Indiana where they obtained their marriage license. From there, they drove to Toledo, Ohio and were married in a large Lutheran Church near downtown, with Dad's Mom and his sister Ellen as their witnesses. They had accompanied them that morning when they set out to "tie the knot". Mom and Dad both enjoyed having a good time at Saturday night dance halls and "on the town" in Toledo. It just seems natural that they would find each other and get married one day, even though neither of their families originally thought it was a good idea. With "The Great Depression" in full swing, they had to know it wouldn't be easy for them. Following are some pictures of Mom when she was a young woman, as well as a picture of Dad in his wild "single" days.

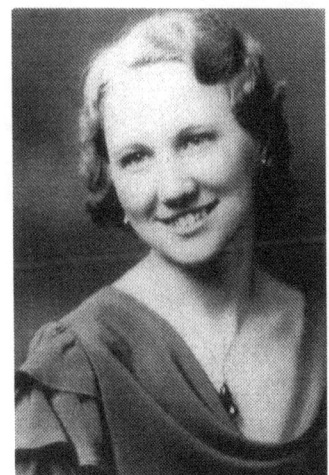
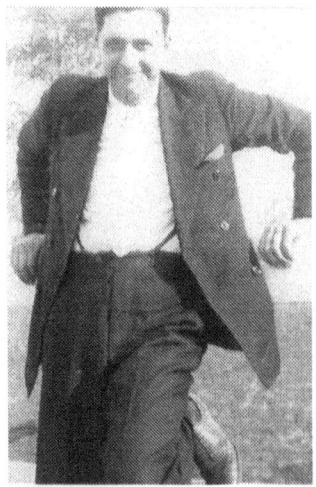
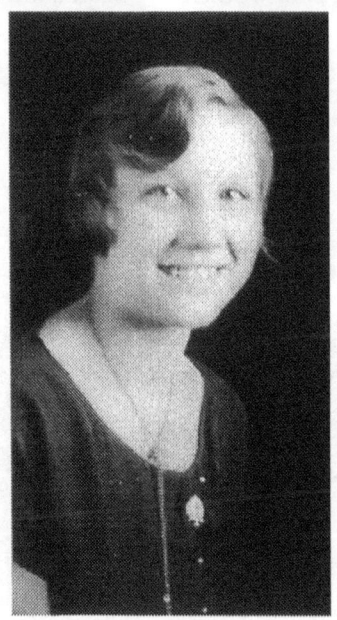

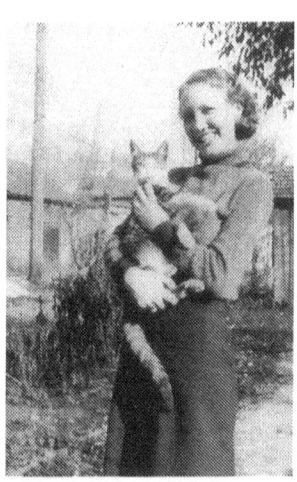

Their first child, Patricia Ann, was born on September 25, 1936. The following picture was taken when she was just an infant. Dad would have been about 27 and Mom would have been 23 at this time.

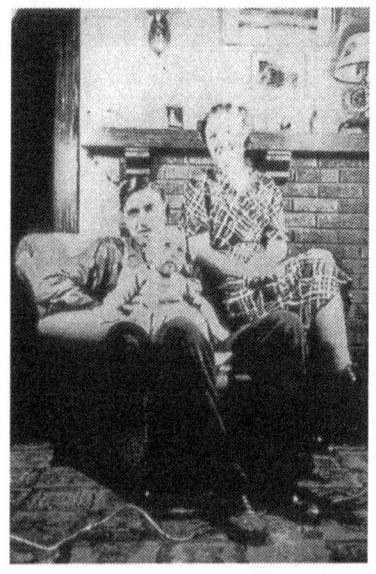

Dad, Mom, and Pat, around 1937

IN THE BEGINNING

Of course, I definitely don't remember the day that I was born, but Mom told me about the "blessed event" many times. I was born on September 30, 1939 in the little town of Petersburg, Michigan, near the tail-end of the Depression.

Since money was tight, they decided to have me at home, so I was born at the house at 83 W. Vesey Street in Petersburg, where Mom and Dad lived almost all of 56 married years together. Back then, it was not the least bit uncommon for women to give birth at home. According to Mom, when she went into labor, her sister, Edna, came over to the house and Doc Smith and his nurse arrived later for the delivery. Apparently, I decided to come into the world feet first and was very stubborn about taking my first breath. So while Doc Smith attended to Mom, he instructed his nurse give me a shot of something to jump-start my heart, and Mom and Dad named me Kay Jean.

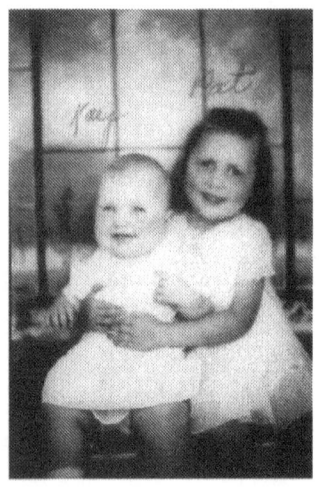 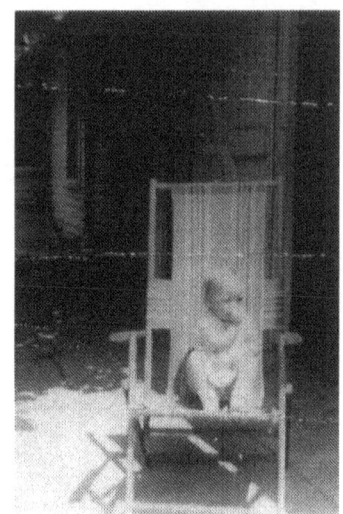

Kay and Pat, around 1940   **Kay**

When I was about 21 months old I got a little brother. Mom decided to stay home for this delivery, too, and this time all went well. My new brother, John Robert, was born June 27, 1941, and named after our grandfathers, John Gaertner and Robert Redick.

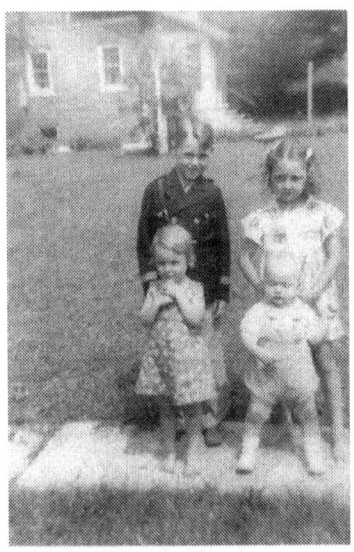

Glen Allen, Pat, Kay, and John

I was too young to remember the attack on Pearl Harbor in 1941; however, I remember the "blackouts" we had in Petersburg later on. When the fire siren blew, everyone was supposed to turn off all their lights and wait for the "all clear" before turning them back on. If your lights were accidentally on, one of the local "Air Raid Wardens" would come to the door to remind you to turn them off. I remember thinking we had to be very quiet so the "enemy" wouldn't hear us.

Mom and Dad also took us to see some mock battle scenes that were depicted with mannequins dressed in American, German, and Japanese uniforms. We also stood on bleachers and watched a staged battle on a field, complete with tanks and loud explosions.

Since John and I were so close in age, there was the usual sibling rivalry and we had our share of "disagreements," two of which resulted in permanent scars for both of us. We always had a lot of fun jumping on our beds (as if they were trampolines), and playing in mud puddles after a good rain was lots of fun, too.

As a matter of fact, those mud puddles got John and me in trouble with our next door neighbor. It seems one day after playing in some mud puddles, we decided to dry off on her sheets that were hanging on her clothesline. At the time, it seemed like the logical thing to do so Mom wouldn't get mad. I guess John and I had a lot of fun till the neighbor saw us and came storming over to the house and told Mom. Now, back in the early 1940's, doing laundry wasn't as easy as it is today. It involved using a "wringer" washing machine and usually two rinse tubs, all of which had to be filled with hot and cold water, most likely with a bucket. If anyone remembers the wringer washing machine, to a child, it looked like a pretty dangerous "household appliance." Needless to say, when Mom was doing laundry I kept my distance, lest I get my arm caught in the wringer clean up to my shoulder. In fact, I had seen things (like socks and washcloths) wrapped so tightly around the wringer, Mom had to hit the release bar on the wringer really hard to free them. Pretty scary! She also had a washboard that she used with a bar of Fels Naptha soap to scrub out stubborn stains. Anyway, the last thing I remember after the neighbor went back home was Mom chasing John and me toward our outhouse. We ran in and locked the door, but I doubt that saved us from the spanking we so deserved.

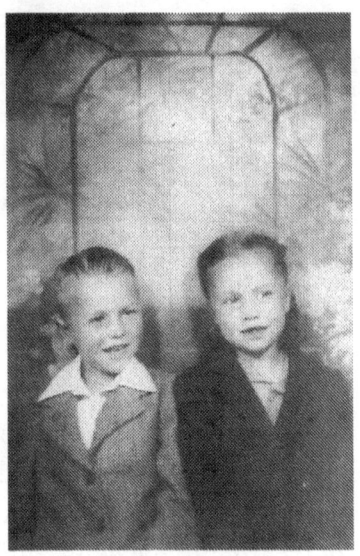

John and Kay

I'll never forget the aviator hat John loved to wear. Even though it came down over his ears, he wore it in all kinds of weather and it wouldn't surprise me in the least if I heard he even wore it to bed. He eventually traded it for a baseball cap. I probably should have known that one day, after he was discharged from the Navy, John would actually get his pilot's license and have his own plane.

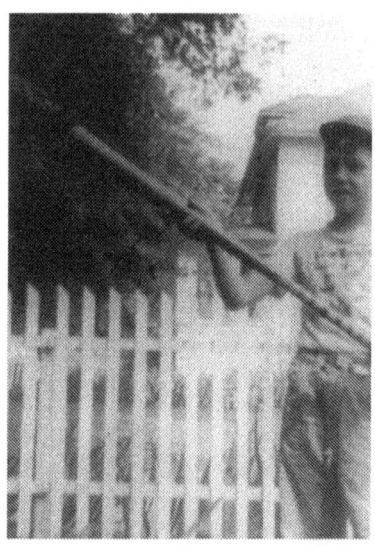

John

We lived in a three-bedroom house on the corner of Vesey Street and Davis Street, situated on a large double lot. It was painted white and had a porch with a railing that ran the full length of the front of the house, and had a trellis covered with red roses in the summer on the east side. We also had a "wood shed" directly behind the house with grape vines growing on the east side of the shed, as well as two chicken coops and an outhouse beyond that. Red and black raspberry bushes grew along the back property line, and Dad always had a garden on the east side of the house. As our family grew, so did the size of (and the need for) the garden. Dad planted strawberries, as well as all kinds of vegetables that he and Mom canned. He even planted potatoes that he put in a potato bin in the basement when they were ready. Dad always had a neat garden and worked hard to keep the weeds out. Despite all of Dad's weeding, every once in a while, during the summer, we'd see Grandpa Gaertner hoeing out in the garden early in the morning. It probably had as much to do with Grandpa not having anything better to do now that he was retired from farming as it had to do with there actually being weeds in the garden.

Mom and Dad both enjoyed bowling and managed to get out one night a week to bowl with friends at the bowling alley in Dundee. They bowled in separate leagues, and one night they went to an exhibition put on by a "trick" bowler named Andy Veripapa. I know they were very impressed because that was just about all they could talk about the next morning. They also enjoyed getting together with friends on Saturday nights to play their favorite card game, Euchre. Dad was one of those persons who really took his games seriously and always remembered every card that had been played.

Dad was also on the finance committee at our Church, as well as a member of the Petersburg Volunteer Fire Department. In fact, the firemen also served as Peace Officers in the village for a while and had to take turns evenings keeping an eye on things. Much to their relief, the village eventually hired a constable full time.

Mom's parents, Robert and Ella Redick, lived in Petersburg on the other side of town. Grandma was a great cook (everyone loved her homemade noodles) and she made a maraschino cherry layer cake with a fluffy icing that was out of this world. Another one of her specialties was the divinity candy she made each year at Christmas time. She liked to crochet in her spare time, and I remember she had a canary in a cage in the dining room that "sang" along with the radio. She always made sure whenever one of us was sick to bring us our very own jar of strawberry jam to "help us get better." They had a garden behind their house where they grew some of their vegetables, as well as some of grandma's favorite flowers.

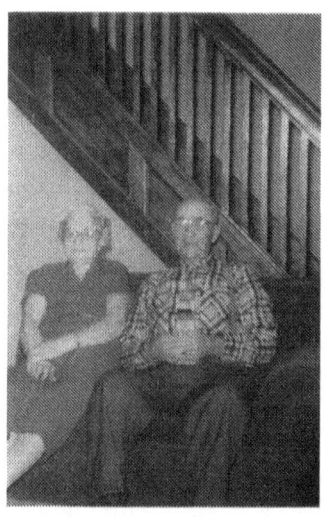

Grandma and Grandpa Redick

Grandma's father (and our Great Grandfather), Grandpa Larkin, lived with them and slept in an upstairs bedroom. I was so young at the time, that I barely remember him. However, when he passed away in his bedroom, I overheard someone saying they had brought him downstairs on a stretcher. At that point in my young life, the only "stretcher" I was familiar with was the one Mom used to stretch her lace curtains on when she washed them. I was quite puzzled as to why they'd have to bring him down on a curtain stretcher, but not quite brave enough to ask anyone why.

Grandpa worked for the railroad and stopped over to see us whenever he could, sometimes bringing us a surprise. In fact when I'd shown an interest in learning to twirl a baton, he brought one over for me.

Pat and I would take turns staying overnight with Grandma and Grandpa, and it seemed like the spare bedroom we slept in was always cold! Still, we never turned down the chance to stay overnight and get the extra attention they always gave us.

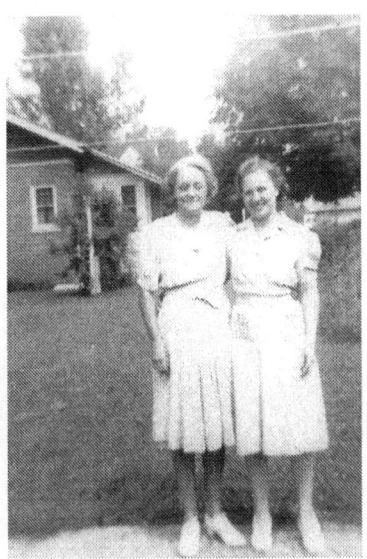

Grandma Redick and Mom

Dad's parents, John and Anna Gaertner, lived in the country, about two miles north of town on Petersburg Road (at one time actually known as Gaertner Road). Going out to their farm was almost always an adventure. Grandpa farmed his land with horse and plow, and he also had a few cows he milked. If we went out to the barn when he was doing chores, he'd give us fresh milk and sometimes we'd use the cup to drink water from an outside pump they had. (This was also a treat, since Petersburg had sulfur water and Grandpa had well water on the farm.) He had a corn sheller and a grinding wheel we liked to play with and chasing their chickens around the yard usually resulted in us stepping in something unpleasant - chances were, if it was summer - we were barefoot. They also had plenty of wild daisies growing around their yard in the summer that we'd pick for Mom and Grandma.

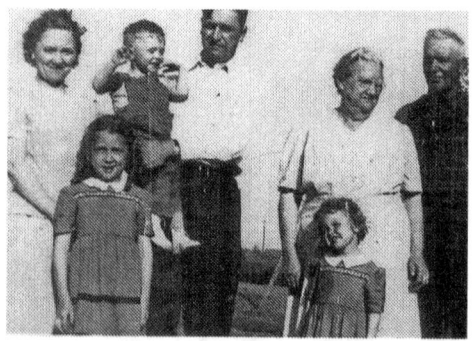

Gaertner clan, around 1943

Grandma Gaertner did all her cooking on a wood stove and we always knew she'd have homemade bread and soft sugar cookies for us to eat whenever we went to see her. She was also a huge Detroit Tiger fan and listened to their games without fail on the radio. Grandpa had a Model T with a rumble seat in back, and if we were really good he'd take us for a ride down the road and back. I remember Grandma standing out in the yard and watching us the entire time to make sure we didn't stand up while going down the road. If we spent the night at their house, we'd sleep upstairs in a soft feather bed covered with a hand-made quilt.

I remember one summer when the guys in the family, uncles and cousins, got together to help Grandpa bale hay to put up in the barn. Grandpa's horses pulled the hay wagon while the guys stacked the bales on it. I was even lucky enough to get a ride on the wagon, but only after I had managed to step on a few sand burrs with my bare feet. You can be sure, that Grandma would always put on "quite a feed" for everyone when their work was finished.

We attended St Peter's Lutheran Church in Petersburg, where we also went to Sunday school. Later on, we attended Catechism classes and after Confirmation, became communicant members of the Church. Pat and I went a couple of years to their little one-room school house next door. I went there for first and second grade. Grandpa and Grandma Redick's house was close enough to the school that sometimes we'd take the lunches

Mom sent with us to their house and have lunch with Grandma. We also went to their Vacation Bible School in the summer.

AFTER THE WAR

Early in 1946, Grandma Gaertner passed away quite suddenly of a heart attack. By then, Mom had found out she was expecting another baby, but never got the chance to tell Grandma the good news. Grandpa eventually sold his farm and moved into a smaller house in Petersburg near Aunt Ellen Kampmueller, Dad's sister. She was a large, affectionate woman who was an excellent cook and who always had a smile and some sort of treats for us. It was always special for us to visit Aunt Ellen and her husband, Uncle Fred. They had three children, a son Carl who was away at college another son Tom who had also graduated from school and had a job. They also had a daughter JoAnn, who was still in high school.

Our brother, James Lester, was born August 29, 1946. Dad hired a local lady, Mrs. Harwick, to take care of us until our Mom and new little brother came home from the hospital. It was early in September when they came home, and by then we were back in school (I was in third grade). I remember coming home from school, walking in the back door and seeing him for the first time. He was asleep in a crib in the dining room and looked so tiny. He had really fine, blond hair, and I remember Mom telling us to be quiet so we didn't wake him. We all absolutely adored him and loved playing with him and making him laugh.

Dear Mama
How are you and baby brother? We are lonesome to see you. Mrs. Harwick reads to us. She gave me a dime for helping her. I got some pop with it.
Love
Kay Jean

Before he started walking, he had a rather unique way of getting around. Instead of creeping on his hands and knees, he sort of hopped along on his bottom. At other times, he would slide around the floor on an old pie tin that we placed under his bottom. When he was still little, we gave him the nickname "Lovey Dovey," and later shortened it to "Dovey." In fact, John also had a nickname; we called him "John Boy" (and that was many years before the name was popularized on "The Waltons" TV series).

In the fall we looked forward to Halloween and trick or treating, and would always have a lot of fun going from door to door, while people tried to guess who we were before giving us our "treat." The only bad part about trick or treating was the uncomfortable masks we had to wear back then. Not only were they hard to breathe in, they were difficult to see out of as well. But what the heck, we were getting candy, popcorn, and all sorts of goodies and it made it all worth while. Halloween was also the time when you might wake up the next morning and find your windows soaped (or waxed!) or worse yet, find your outhouse tipped over. Also in the fall, when the leaves started dropping from the trees we'd get out the rakes, rake them into a big pile and take turns jumping into it, and usually the neighborhood kids would join in. When we were done playing, Dad would rake them to the side of the street to burn, and if we had any apples or, better yet, on rare occasions, marshmallows, we'd roast them over the fire.

Large family get-togethers such as Thanksgiving were usually at Grandpa and Grandma Redick's house. Then, after Thanksgiving, we'd start memorizing our parts (usually Bible verses) for the Christmas Eve program, and going back to the church on Sunday afternoons to practice for an hour or two. When he was a small child, John had a beautiful voice. However, Pat and I were absolutely horrified when he said he'd volunteered to sing a solo one Christmas Eve. As it turned out, the song was beautiful and he made the whole family very proud of him.

After we finished the church program on Christmas Eve, we'd go home and hurry off to bed before Santa got there. According to Pat, one Christmas Eve on the way home,

Dad said he saw Santa and his sleigh on a roof the other side of town. She said we hid in the back seat on the floor of the car and ran straight up to bed when we got home. Manys the Christmas Eve I lay in bed, eyes closed (pretending to be asleep) and listening for sleigh bells. One Christmas morning Dad "found" a gift in the yard that he said had fallen from Santa's sleigh when he flew over the night before.

John got an erector set one year that provided many hours of entertainment for both he and Dad. It had a small "motor" and they built all sorts of contraptions and structures. And one more thing...Santa always remembered to leave something new for the train set that Dad put up around the tree each year. And speaking of Christmas trees, Dad preferred a short-needled pine tree, and it had to be "the perfect" tree. If a Christmas tree had a bare spot, most people would just turn that spot toward the wall. Not Dad! He'd get out his hand drill and hacksaw and do a "makeover" on the tree. He'd drill a hole in the bare spot on the trunk and insert one of the spare branches that he'd sawed from the base of the tree. He was just as particular about the way he trimmed the tree, and it always looked great. He used three different kinds of lights on the tree, but my favorite ones were the bubble lights. Dad also had some beautiful hand blown glass ornaments from Germany on the tree that had belonged to his Mom and Dad, and would finish by decorating the tree with tinsel. He also had red cellophane wreaths he put in the windows. Usually during the Holiday season, Dad would take us to Toledo to see how some of the homes were decorated in Ottawa Hills and other more affluent parts of the city. I guess his love of Christmas must have rubbed off on me, because the Holidays are also my favorite time of the year.

The rest of the winter we played outside a lot, sledding, ice-skating and building snowmen. I remember Dad ice skating on "Dead River" and pulling us behind on a sled. Dead River is a small tributary of the Raisin River, which runs through Petersburg. Just north of town, Dead River is most likely where Dad learned to skate as a young man. A few years later, we had our own ice-skating "rink" that drew most of the neighborhood kids. Once Mom and Dad were finished with the garden in the fall, Dad would bank the dirt up around the edge and flood it when the temperature started to drop. Since Dad belonged to the Fire Department, they brought one of the trucks over to flood our garden on a couple of different occasions.

In the winter, we heated our house with a coal furnace that had one large register in the dining room for the entire house. Mom usually had her rocking chair near the register, and that was my most favorite place when I came in from outside to get warm. Also, when Mom did the laundry in the winter, she'd dry some of the clothes on a wooden rack next to the register. She dried the rest of them on some clothes lines that were strung across the basement.

There was no such thing as a multivitamin when I was a kid; instead, we had to take some cod liver oil! Every day, without fail, Mom would call us out into the kitchen and give each of us a spoonful of the stuff. When we happened to come down with a cold, Mom was also very liberal with Vicks. If we had a sore throat or chest cold, she would slather the Vicks on our throat and chest; warm a flannel cloth in the oven or over the dining room register, then safety pin the warm cloth around our neck before we went to bed. I'm not sure it really worked, but it sure felt good. Another "cure" for the common cold was to put some Vicks in a little water, heat it on the stove, and then have us breathe the vapors. And although I don't remember having the mumps or chicken pox, I do remember the measles. I spent several days, for the most part quarantined in my bedroom, with a blanket over the window to shut out the light.

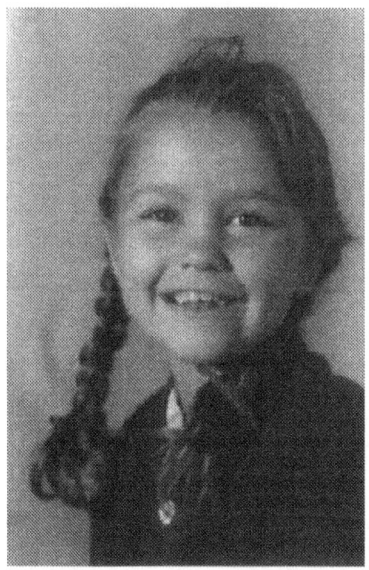

Kay, around 1946

In the spring, Pat and I would go shopping with Mom in Toledo for new dresses and hats to wear to Church on Easter Sunday. We would sometimes go shopping in Adrian or Monroe, but being from a small town, going shopping in Toledo was something we'd always look forward to. We'd go to Tiedke's, a store in downtown Toledo, and we'd always get soft serve ice cream cones and ride the escalator. I can still remember the cylinders into which the cashiers would place the money for a purchase, and send it on its way. Moments later, the change would magically return to the cashier in the cylinder. It's similar to the system still used by bank cashiers at drive-thru windows.

The night before Easter, we'd make little nests out of grass for the Easter bunny and line them up along the front porch railing. When we woke up the next morning we'd find colored eggs in the nests and baskets of candy in the living room. Also, Dad would sometimes take us with him in the spring when he went hunting for mushrooms in the woods. But instead of hunting for mushrooms, we kids spent our time swinging from the wild grape vines in the trees and picking wild flowers to take back home to Mom. I hate to think of how many mushrooms we probably trampled before Dad could get to them. He also liked driving along country roads in the spring looking for asparagus. It sounds unusual, but it was quite common back then. Most of the time, he'd drive along Deerfield Road between Petersburg and Adrian, and look for it along the railroad tracks. Then when we'd get near Adrian, we'd cross a bridge that we called the "bumpity bump bridge" because of the noise it made when Dad drove over it.

In the summertime, most Sunday afternoons after we'd finished dinner dishes we'd go for a ride, and usually wind up stopping somewhere along the way for ice cream cones. One time after we'd finished our cones, Dad asked, "Who's ready for another cone?" Needless to say, he didn't have to ask us a second time and we couldn't believe our good luck. Sometimes, instead of having dinner at home after Church, we'd take a picnic to the beach at Wamplers Lake in the Irish Hills. Other times, we'd visit friends or relatives for a while. Dad took us to "hot rod" races, county fairs or carnivals, and every 4th of July we'd go to the Dundee carnival to see the fireworks. Occasionally we'd see the fireworks in Monroe first and stop in Dundee on the way home to watch their fireworks. Because he was a truck driver, I guess Dad never tired of driving. As a result, we got to see more of southern Michigan than some of our friends did.

We could always find something to do at home in the summer, as well. One of our favorite things was pitching a tent in the backyard and pretending we were camping. Mom had a couple of old army blankets she'd let us toss over the clothesline and secure with some wooden clothespins. There was an older couple who lived in the house behind us and although they didn't have any children of their own, they had a huge swing in their front yard for the neighborhood kids to play on. It was suspended by four cables from a big limb in a tree and the seat was large enough to accommodate at least six kids. We took turns pushing each other on it and as long as we behaved ourselves and dressed properly (no shorts, it was against her religion) we could play on the swing whenever we wanted. Sometimes we'd go across the street to play with the kids next door. However, our street wasn't paved back then, and the village would spray oil on it to keep down the dust. Mom would take Dad's shovel, get some dirt from the garden and make a path for us to use when we crossed the street. We usually played outside barefoot in the summer, and somehow, every once in a while, we'd managed to stray a little off the path Mom had made for us. As a result, Mom would wind up having to scrub oil off the bottoms of our feet anyway.

There was a man who delivered ice around town to those who still used ice boxes for their food instead of refrigerators. Each homeowner had a card they displayed in a window for the iceman, to let him know how many pounds of ice they needed. If it was a hot day he'd sometimes chip off some ice for us to chew on while we played, and quite often it was so covered with sawdust, we'd have to wipe it on our clothes first. I guess you could call him a 1940's version of the Good Humor man. In addition to the iceman, there was also the Sealtest milkman who delivered dairy products, a dry cleaner who picked up and dropped off your dry cleaning, and even a bread man. Very few families had two cars, so there was a real need for these types of home delivery services.

Every summer there was a man who came to town and went door-to-door sharpening scissors and knives. He'd sit on the porch steps while he worked, and we'd watch him through the screen door. Because one of his legs was actually a "peg leg" (sort of like a pirate) we were quite curious as we watched him through the screen door, but still kept our distance. Later, we learned that he was what was called a "hobo" back then. Perhaps he had ridden into town on one of the trains that used to pass through town daily. Today, the trains no longer run through Petersburg and the tracks have long since been removed.

Of course, when we were children, we always had some sort of pet to play with - usually a dog. We had a couple of dachshunds named Gretel and Brownie, and later on a beagle named Cleo. Gretel was our "bad dog" who was always getting into something. One year she knocked over our Christmas tree three times, breaking some of Dad's glass ornaments. Another time, Pat and I got matching wine-colored chenille bath robes and matching slippers trimmed with white rabbit fur for Christmas. While we were at Grandma and Grandpa's having dinner, Gretel chewed all the fur off of one of Pat's slippers, as well as chewing the arm off the doll she got for Christmas, too. Oh, she was one busy dog!

Although Cleo was a registered beagle, and supposedly a hunting dog, she spent the winter months indoors when it was too cold for her in her home in the shed. She wasn't a bad hunting dog, but if you weren't careful, she was inclined to get on the scent of a rabbit or pheasant and just keep running. In the winter, her favorite place was perched on the back of the sofa where she could look out the living room window. In the summer months, she would stay in her shed, which also had a small fenced in area for her. The fence wasn't so much to keep her in as it was to keep the male dogs in the neighborhood at a distance from her. It seems Cleo suffered from poor morals when it came to these matters.

We also had a parakeet named Joey. However, one morning, Mom found him on the bottom of his cage, and had to deliver the sad news to us that he'd passed away. When our friends from next door heard about it and came over to offer their condolences, we decided to have a funeral. Our friend, David conducted the funeral - a Catholic service, and we buried Joey next to a maple tree in the back yard.

Mom and Dad raised chickens in the two coops behind the house, and one summer we kids "adopted" one of Mom's chickens and named her Henrietta. We dressed her in some of our doll clothes and pushed her around the neighborhood in one of our doll buggies. Later on, when Mom and Dad had decided to quit raising chickens, they cleaned up one of the chicken coops and let us use it for a playhouse. Actually, it was sort of the neighborhood "clubhouse".

Since Mom liked writing poetry and jingles, every once in a while she would enter a contest. One time she entered a contest that was advertised on the Bob Hope radio show, sponsored by Pepsodent. She drew a picture of Bob Hope using the letters in Pepsodent in the caricature, and if I remember correctly, it was a very good likeness of him. In fact, so good that we were sure she'd probably win the contest. We were all pretty disappointed when she didn't win. Not even Honorable Mention! A few years later, she actually won a prize for a jingle she entered in a contest on The Arthur Godfrey Show. The prize was called "an automatic dishwasher," but in truth, it amounted to little more than a fancy sprayer for a kitchen sink. The sprayer had a foaming brush handle for cleaning the dishes. Unfortunately, it was a little too modern for our old sink and just collected dust for several years. I think Mom wound up giving it away.

OUR FAMILY'S FIRST BIG SETBACK

Every family faces its own tests over the years. In late summer of 1947, we had our own. Mom became so ill she was confined to bed, and I suppose at the time they thought she probably had the flu. Aunt Edna lived nearby and checked on her occasionally while Dad was at work to see if she needed anything. However, one afternoon when she stopped by, Mom seemed to have taken a turn for the worse and Aunt Edna called the doctor. By the time we got home from school that afternoon, there was an ambulance in front of our house and they were preparing to take Mom to a hospital. Back then, the ambulance was also used as a hearse for funerals. I didn't see Dad when I first got there, and when I went looking for him I found him outside the back door, crying.

Mom was taken to a hospital in Toledo and our family was split up temporarily when Pat, John, Jim and I went to stay with relatives of Mom and Dad. Pat went to stay with Grandpa and Grandma Redick, and John stayed with Uncle Louis and Aunt Leona, Dad's brother and sister-in-law. I went to stay with Aunt Ellen and Uncle Fred, Dad's sister and brother-in-law. Our little brother, Jim, went to stay with Mom's sister and brother-in-law, Catherine and Glen, in Ann Arbor while she took a couple of weeks off work. When she went back to work, he went to stay with John at Uncle Louis and Aunt Leona's.

Mom was at the hospital in Toledo for a short time. Then she was transferred to the University of Michigan Hospital in Ann Arbor and placed in a separate building that specialized in contagious illnesses. It was after she was admitted there that we learned she had polio. It seems even though our country was in the midst of a polio epidemic, nobody had thought a small town housewife whose main interests were her family and home would be exposed to the disease. They later came to the conclusion she may have been exposed to it when she and Dad went to an Air Show shortly before she became ill. Once it got around town that our Mom had polio, and nobody was really sure what caused it, we kids were somewhat "shunned" at school. Although John and I were too young to notice, Pat was especially aware of the way some of her classmates avoided her. This was because not only did polio cause paralysis, it could sometimes be fatal.

While Mom was confined to the hospital in Ann Arbor, Dad would drive from Petersburg to work in Toledo each morning. After work, he'd return home and then make the long drive to Ann Arbor. Back then, there were no expressways, just a two lane road that went through the towns of Dundee and Milan on the way to Ann Arbor. Poor Dad was quite the trooper. I'm sure it had to be a terrible strain on him, emotionally, physically, and financially, to keep our family together. When he could find time, he'd try to stop by and see us, and one weekend he took Pat, John and I to the hospital to see Mom. We thought we'd actually get to see her and talk to her, but as it turned out, we stood outside on a porch and waved to her through a window. The polio had affected her hands, arms, shoulders and also her breathing and swallowing. They even had an iron lung outside her door just in case she would need it. Since Mom's sister and brother-in-law, Catherine and Glen, both worked at the hospital and lived nearby, they would stop in and check on her each day, too.

Staying with Aunt Ellen and Uncle Fred was quite something. They lived in a large house a few blocks from our house and I slept alone in an upstairs bedroom. Since I was a really finicky eater, Aunt Ellen tried to fix foods I'd like, as well as making hot cocoa for my breakfast or bedtime treat. My cousin, JoAnn, was in high school and a Varsity cheerleader. So that meant we went to all the "home" basketball games - something I'd never done before. (Eventually, JoAnn told me she had a confession to make. She said she had to admit, when I came to stay with them she was more than a little jealous of all the attention I got).

As Christmas drew near, I came home from school one day and Aunt Ellen told me Dad had stopped by and left a dress for me to wear in the Christmas Eve program at church. It was dark blue velvet and had a white lace collar. It was the prettiest dress I'd ever seen, but when I tried it on, Aunt Ellen said it was too big and Dad would have to take it back. Well, I started crying and when I got a tear on it, she decided to alter it so it would fit me. A few days before Christmas, Aunt Ellen took me up town with her to run some errands. When I found a five dollar bill on the sidewalk, I felt like the richest kid in the world. It was the most money I'd ever held in my hand. And since I'd wanted to get gifts for my family for Christmas, she took me to the local variety store to do my shopping. I managed to find gifts for everyone in the family with that five dollars, and she wrapped them for me. It's possible that Aunt Ellen "planted" that money for me to find, but I'll never know. As Christmas drew near, one day at school the teacher asked each child in my class what they wanted for Christmas. I remember saying I wanted my Mom to come home for Christmas. Although Aunt Ellen and the rest of the family did all they could to make my stay with them comfortable, I desperately missed being at home with my family.

Years later, Mom would often tell us how she'd listen to the radio while in the hospital and as the Holidays approached, she'd cry each time she'd hear Bing Crosby singing "I'll Be Home for Christmas." Well, she did come home for Christmas! We had Christmas dinner over at Grandma and Grandpa Redick's house, then Mom stayed at their house for two weeks while Dad made arrangements for all of us to come back home again. Mom's youngest sister, Roberta, and her husband, Gabe, lived nearby and she helped Grandma take care of Mom. To this day, each time I hear the song "I'll Be Home for Christmas," I think of Mom. It must have been a terrible time for her.

We all went back home to stay after Dad hired a young woman named Donna to help out around the house. She lived with us during the week and helped out with the cooking, cleaning, and laundry. She was with us for a while and after she left we got another "hired girl," Juanita. One evening after supper Juanita told Pat and me she'd give us a dime if we'd do the dishes. Since ten cents went a lot further back then, we agreed. Well, after we'd finished the dishes, and went to collect our money, she said we had to split the ten cents and gave us each a nickel. We'd been had! Not long after that, Dad and Mom decided we didn't need a housekeeper and we all pitched in to get things done around the house. Of course, Pat and I did the dishes, as well as doing the sweeping and dusting. Dad did whatever he could when he got home from work and on his days off. As we got older, Pat and I would "draw lots" on Saturday mornings to decide which rooms we each had to clean that day.

During this time, Mom was going to a clinic in Toledo each week for therapy on her arms and hands to, hopefully, regain some strength again. She was also given a brace to wear on her right hand and forearm, and needed help with both putting it on, as well as taking it off at the end of the day. In time, she saw it as more of a hindrance rather than something meant to help her, and stopped wearing it altogether. In fact, that's probably the only time I recall seeing Mom have what would now be called a "meltdown" when trying to eat her evening meal while wearing the brace. She became so frustrated she was reduced to tears and left the table. It probably didn't help matters when we kids stared at her while she tried to eat. (Many years later, the University of Michigan Hospital contacted Mom regarding participation in a study of Post-Polio Syndrome. One doctor, in fact, told Mom that they could now perform surgery on her crippled hand that would restore some of its use to her. By this time, Mom was well along in years, suffering with arthritis, and probably had more than her fill of doctors and hospitals. She declined their invitation for the study, as well as for any surgery on her hand).

Pat and I continued doing the dishes just about every night, right up until we left home. We had a radio in the kitchen, and we'd always listen to it while doing the dishes. Sometimes we'd listen to country music on a station out of Cincinnati, Ohio, and the rest of the time we'd listen to the latest songs on CKLW. As a matter of fact, our entire family loved to listen to music, and we even had a radio on which we could cut our own records. Many times when the family got together, Aunts, Uncles and cousins would pass the time harmonizing and singing a lot of the popular old songs. I still have some of the records we made back then, but as far as I know, no way to play them. We had a record of Mom singing "Don't Fence Me In" and one of me singing "Heart Aches" (except I thought the words were "Hard Eggs," so that's the way I sang it). We also had a recording of John singing "I'm a Big Girl Now." I can't imagine how tired he became of hearing about that as he got older. The records we bought to play on our record player ranged from organ music to current popular songs or Spike Jones.

Meanwhile, Mom was determined to see things return to, at the least, near normal again. She eventually managed to cook, do some light house cleaning and with Dad's help, the laundry. She learned to use her (treadle) sewing machine again, as well as learning to crochet. She was also an avid reader and loved to do crossword puzzles. Although Mom had very limited use of her arms and hands, I never heard her complain about her disability. If she wanted to do something, she was always very determined and usually found a way to accomplish it. However, one of Mom's biggest challenges was trying to write again, since she had to hold the pen in her right hand and guide it along with her left hand. As a result,

Dad took over the task of mailing out the Birthday and Christmas cards and all other correspondence.

Mom told me many years later that when she was released from University Hospital, her doctor told her she'd have to undergo months of therapy on her arms and hands. To which she replied, "Will I be able to play the piano?" When the doctor replied, "Absolutely", she said, "Good, I've always wanted to play the piano!" The amazing thing about Mom was, with all the pain and frustration she had endured, she never lost her sense of humor and always liked to hear a good joke (or tell one).

Around 1949, Dad started taking us on summer vacations. Our first one was up north to a hunting lodge near Hillman, Michigan with friends of Mom and Dad. Even though we stayed at the lodge we were sort of roughing it, as there was no electricity or running water. We all slept in a large bedroom that was furnished with double bunk beds. There was a "dump" near the woods behind the lodge, and an old outhouse near the dump. It just so happened that bears would come out of the woods sometimes at night and scavenge for food in the dump. Well, Mom was afraid to go out to the outhouse alone at night, so Dad would accompany her when nature called. One night while she and Dad were inside the outhouse, the floor collapsed under their combined weight, leaving them with a few scratches and a good deal of embarrassment. Dad and his friend spent the next day of our vacation putting a new floor in the outhouse.

Dad and his friend, Bob, also went fishing at a small lake nearby called Fletcher's Pond while we were staying at the lodge, and some evenings we'd pile into the car and go out "shining " deer. Back in the "good old days" we only saw deer when we went up north vacationing. However, now it's quite common to see deer locally just about anywhere in the area, even within the city limits where they live in the parks and nearby woods.

THE 1950'S: LIFE RETURNS TO NORMAL

Soon, Dad started working all the overtime he could at the dairy. He also worked at his brother Louie's gas station on his days off from the dairy, as well as weekends and evenings. I remember Dad saving all his dimes in a jar so he could go up to northern Michigan deer hunting with his brother-in-law, Fred, and his nephews. They stayed at a farmhouse near Glennie, owned by a woman named Edna, who made extra money during the deer hunting season by renting rooms to the hunters. The money they paid for their room also included their meals. Over the years that followed, Dad went hunting up north with a good friend from Toledo, Louie Vortebruggen, with whom he had worked at Sealtest Dairy. Many years later, he went hunting with Pat's husband, Earl, and even John and Jim went with him for a couple of years. I think he really enjoyed the chance to get away and just be with the guys. Coming home with a deer was not really that important to him.

When it came to shopping for groceries, Dad bought most of our groceries in Toledo. And because he worked for the dairy delivering products to some of the larger stores in Toledo, he knew where he could get the best bargains. He and Mom would plan the menu for the week, and he'd shop after he got out of work on his pay day. I always loved watching Dad unload the grocery bags when he got home - He had a "sweet tooth" like me and usually threw in a few packages of candy and store-bought cookies that weren't on the list. I remember some of his favorites were circus peanuts and chocolate peanut clusters. We also bought some of our groceries at a store in Petersburg that was owned by Mom's brother-in-law Glen Breitner, Aunt Edna's husband.

Most of my friends were kids who lived within about two blocks of our house. In the summertime, we'd get together and play Red Rover or Hide and Seek. We also played a game called "Eenie Eye Over," which involved tossing a ball over the roof of our wood shed to a person on the other side who had to catch the ball. If we could get enough kids together, we'd choose sides and play softball or football. When Mom turned the porch light on, that was our signal to come inside. Later on, when Pat and I were old enough to start dating, it was the signal that we'd sat out in the driveway long enough, and it was time to come inside.

I had a friend, Mary, who lived in Monroe and would spend the summer with her aunt and uncle who lived next door. They owned one of the bars uptown and occasionally Mary would have to walk uptown to talk to them about one thing or another. I was allowed to walk uptown, but absolutely forbidden to go into the bar. So once in a while, as I waited outside for her, I'd try to look inside the door to see just what, exactly, was going on in there. The smell of beer and smoke drifted out the door, and I could hear the jukebox playing, but it was so dark inside I couldn't see a thing. But orders were orders, so I never set foot in the bar.

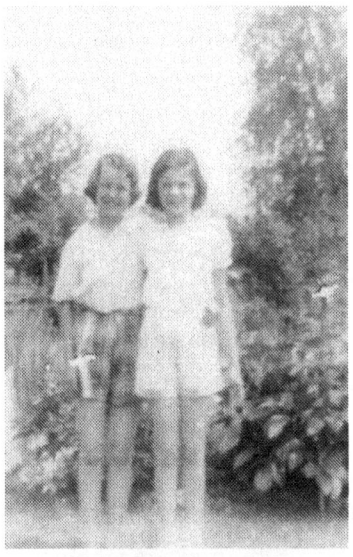

Kay and Mary

Sometimes we'd walk to a small gas station a couple of blocks from our house if we had a little spending money. A bottle of root beer pop cost less than ten cents (and that included the two cent deposit). For another five cents, you could buy an ice cream "dixie cup" and have enough for two root beer floats! And there really was such a thing as penny candy! Another favorite was little candies glued to paper strips, called "dots." I hate to think of how much paper we consumed trying to get that darned candy off the paper! Eventually, Mary's Aunt and Uncle moved to a house on the other side of town and she stopped coming to Petersburg for her summer vacations. We wrote letters for a while, but eventually lost touch with each other.

I had a pair of roller skates that Mom and Dad had bought for me, and how I loved them! They were the kind that clamped onto the soles of my shoes and I used a "key" to adjust them so they fit. We didn't have a sidewalk on our side of the street, so I'd skate back and forth on the sidewalk across from our house. Mom complained about the skates pulling the soles off my shoe. Once I'd learned to skate well enough, I'd go with friends from school or the youth group at Church to the London Skating Rink north of Dundee, near the little town of Azalia.

By now, we had gotten our first television set, and were actually the first family in the neighborhood to get one. Of course, it was black and white and there really wasn't much to watch. It had only a few channels and they all "signed off" at midnight with the Star Spangled Banner. In the morning, before the programming started back up for the day, there would be a "test pattern" of an Indian's head on the screen. Another thing I remember about the television - when the picture got "snowy," Dad had to go outside and turn the pole that supported our roof antenna until the picture cleared up. It was rarely turned on during the day and we'd watch it together in the evening until "soap operas" started. Then, Mom would watch her favorite, "Search for Tomorrow," faithfully every day. Eventually, we'd sit at TV trays, eating supper on Sunday nights while watching Ed Sullivan. They also had wrestling on one night a week, and Grandpa Redick liked to come over to watch that.

Pat got a radio one Christmas and kept it on a small table on her side of the bed, as she had certain programs she liked to listen to before going to sleep at night. However, two of the programs were "Inner Sanctum" and Gang Busters". The first one opened with a slowly squeaking door - too scary for me, and the second opened with the sounds of tires squealing and guns shooting. I remember covering my ears and trying to shut out sounds that scared the heck out of me. Eventually, John made his own "radio", a crystal set that he listened to with earphones. He kept it in his bedroom and occasionally he'd wake up in the morning with indentations on the sides of his head after falling asleep while listening to it. He was also known to read comic books by flashlight after being sent upstairs for bedtime.

Soon we were vacationing every summer at Houghton Lake, near Prudenville. We kids passed the time on the way up north, singing some of our favorites, such as, I've Been Working on the Railroad, a few rounds of Row, Row, Row Your Boat, or songs we'd learned at school. We also read the signs along the road, always hoping to see some Burma Shave signs. I remember one sign that read, "Spring has sprung, the grass has riz, where last year's careless drivers iz." I'm quite sure we didn't have a radio in our car, so this was our only form of entertainment on the long drive. We'd leave early in the morning when we'd set out on our trip, then stop at the city of Clare for lunch along the way. On the way up north, we'd always pass a huge monument with a lumberjack who resembled Paul Bunyan. Whenever we saw that, we knew we were officially "up north."

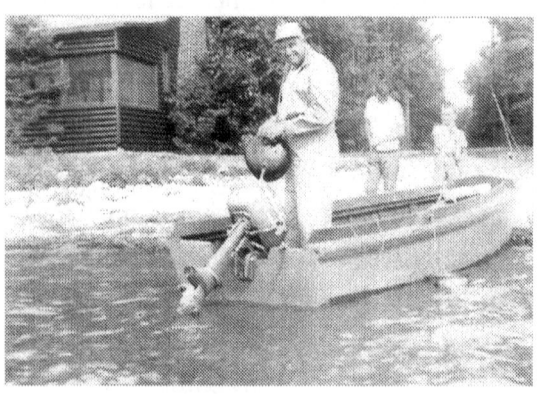

Dad, John, and Jim at Houghton Lake

Mom and Dad liked to rent a lakefront cabin at a couple of different fishing resorts on the North Shore that also included a fishing boat. That way, everyone was happy - Dad could go fishing, and we had a beach to play on and a lake to splash around in. One resort owner's name was Wagner, and they also had a small convenience store a short distance away. The other resort was owned by a family named Moreland. While we were there, Dad would take us on little side trips. One of his favorite places was Reedsburg Dam - another place to fish! We'd also go up to Mackinaw City and take the ferryboat across the Straits. This was before the "Big Mac" bridge was built, and something we always looked forward to. One year, we inadvertently left our little brother, Jim, on the ferry and he came pretty close to taking another round trip on the boat to St. Ignace…this one unplanned.

When Dad got his first car with an automatic shift, we went for a short ride with Grandpa Gaertner in the front seat beside Dad. When we got outside of town, Dad slowed down so Grandpa could "feel" the car shift. Grandpa was amazed (as were we), but he continued to drive his stick shift car until he was well into his 80's and decided to quit driving. I used to hear Mom and Dad talking about the way Grandpa "rode" the clutch. With his engine revving, you could hear him coming a block away. He also had the bad habit of driving straight through four-way stop signs. His reasoning was, "the other car is gonna stop anyway". It was what Grandpa called "a rolling stop." It's amazing that he never smacked into another car.

When I was about 12 years old I started babysitting evenings and weekends. The going rate then was 25 cents an hour and 35 cents after midnight. I used some of my money to buy clothes, records and occasionally a movie magazine. I always knew if I ran into a problem while babysitting, Mom was only a phone call away. And hopefully, so was the telephone operator.

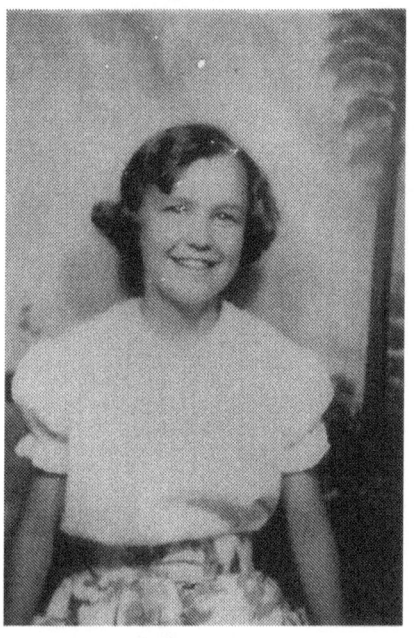

Kay

Our telephone was a wooden box that hung on the north wall in the dining room. It had a mouthpiece on the front to talk into, which you could move up or down to reach the level of your mouth. The handset (receiver) hung from a cradle on the left side of the phone, and when picked up was used for listening to the person at the other end. A small hand crank on the right side was used for calling the operator. We had a party line, which means we shared a phone line with three or four other homeowners. Before turning the crank to reach the operator, we had to listen first to make sure we weren't interrupting someone else's phone call. If the line wasn't busy, we'd turn the crank and when the operator answered, we'd tell her what number we wanted to reach. She'd connect us, using two rows of "cords" she had in front of her, and by ringing the numbers using a hand switch.

Our telephone number was 26F12, which meant one long ring and two short rings. Everyone else on our party line could hear the phone ring and had to determine if it was ringing for them or someone else on the party line, since each home had a distinctive ring pattern. For example, another home might have two long rings. Because we were on a party line, we only used the telephone when it was absolutely necessary, and not without getting Mom or Dad's permission first, so the line wouldn't be tied up. It was also possible for someone on your party line to listen to your calls if they were sneaky enough. How the times have changed!

It took a little longer if we wanted to make a long distance call. After giving the Operator the number we wanted to call, she'd call us back when she had them on the line.

The telephone office was housed in a building in town that also had living quarters for the manager, who had to be available for any calls (incoming or outgoing) during the night. The telephone operator was also the person who "set off" the fire siren in the event of a fire or other emergency.

Our electricity was provided by the Detroit Edison, and they had a building uptown where we paid the monthly bill. They didn't just take the payments; they also gave us free light bulbs when we turned in our bulbs that were broken or burned out. They even repaired small appliances at their "store" or came to your house to repair your electric stove. Now that's service!

Next door to the Edison office was the movie theater that always had a free matinee for the kids at Christmas and Easter. It usually consisted of singing some songs by following the "bouncing ball" on the screen, followed by some cartoons. Dad would also drop us off for the Sunday afternoon matinee once in a while. They'd always have cartoons, or maybe the Three Stooges or Little Rascals before the main movie. There were also newsreels about the recent news events from around the world. I remember some of the movies we saw were "Song of the South," "Bambi" and "The Yearling." And how can I forget the Roy Rogers and Gene Autry westerns we saw, as well as some of our other favorites, Abbott and Costello, Ma and Pa Kettle and the Bowery Boys. When the movie "The Thing" came out, we didn't see it because Mom and Dad thought it was too scary for us. Dundee also had a movie theater and once in a while we'd go there to see a movie that was playing.

When I was in the seventh grade, I took a "musical aptitude test" and we decided I would learn to play the clarinet. We couldn't afford to buy a new one, and since Uncle Louis had a spare one at home (it used to belong to one of his kids) he sold it to Dad. I belonged to the Junior band and took band class at school. I also had homework for band class and my poor family had to put up with all the squeaks and squawks while I practiced at the dining room table. Mom and Dad were very encouraging and went to all my concerts, as well as my impromptu concerts at home when relatives stopped by. It all paid off though, by the time I started my Freshman year in high school I was in the Senior band, played in the marching band at football games, Pep Band at basketball games, parades and concerts. One year our marching band was invited to participate in Band Day at the University of Michigan stadium. As luck would have it, we overslept that morning and I missed the bus. Mom called Grandpa Redick and he came to my rescue. Not only did he take me to the University of Michigan practice field on State Street, he parked his car and enlisted the aid of a band member from the University of Michigan to help me find my own band. I can't remember whether or not Michigan won their game that day. I know I'll never forget the thrill of participating with other high school bands from all over Michigan at half time, so many bands that we covered almost the entire football field. Under the direction of the University of Michigan band director, somehow we managed to pull it all together (even the drums) and play a couple of songs. If I'm not mistaken, that may have been one of the first Band Day's at the University of Michigan.

Pat took Home Economics in high school, and one evening she and some of her classmates decided to prepare something they'd heard about. It was called "pizza pie." Since they had to make everything from scratch, it took most of the evening. So while the dough was rising for the crust, they made the sauce and grated the cheese. Once they put it all together and it was baking in the oven, it smelled absolutely divine. When it was ready, everyone got a piece of it. I have to admit, it was pretty good, even though at that time I wouldn't eat anything that had tomato in it. Who would have thought that pizza would be as popular as it is today? She also had some of her friends over one evening for a Taffy Pull – now THAT looked like a lot of fun. Funny, you never hear of anyone having a taffy pull anymore.

AT LAST! HIGH SCHOOL!

Is it just me, or did the days, weeks, months and years seem to pass by slower than they do now? Of course, the school year always seemed long, but so did our summer vacation. While on vacation, we'd go to the library up town and take out books, which we'd usually read out on our front porch. We were always anxious to go back to school in the fall and see our friends again. Going from eighth grade into (Summerfield) high school was definitely a big change. First of all, I had a locker to keep my books in and a combination I had to remember in order to use the locker. Instead of staying in one classroom for the entire day, we had to go from one classroom to another for different subjects. The classes even seemed to be more difficult, but at least we had a Study Hall so we could get a head start on our homework assignments. We had to get a Pass to go to the restroom and there was a Hallway Monitor to make sure we didn't "goof-off" on our way there. When I was in grade school, I almost always carried a lunch to school. Now that I was in high school I walked home for lunch. Once in a while I bought my lunch at school, or would sometimes walk up town with friends to the local restaurant for a hamburger and a pop.

I made some new friends when I started ninth grade, since some of the kids from around Petersburg went to country schools until they graduated from the eighth grade. I had a couple of friends who lived in the country, and we'd have sleepovers at each other's houses on the weekends. I also had three or four friends who lived in town, and we usually "hung out" around town or at each other's houses on weekends or after school. We had a music store uptown where we'd buy our 45 rpm records and listen to the latest songs. There was even a small clothing store next to the barber shop, and a drug store with an ice cream counter, where we could get a fountain coke or root beer float. For the most part, I pretty much stayed with my small circle of friends throughout high school. It was also around this time that autograph books were popular, and all the girls had to have one. We'd pass them around to all our friends and classmates to sign, and they would usually make up a verse to put in it. I wonder what ever happened to mine! We also kept scrap books with pictures of our friends and various mementos.

Early in 1954 I met a guy from a neighboring town through a friend of mine. He was a couple of years older than I was and went to the same church she did. So until he got his driver's license a couple of months later, we wrote letters and saw each other at his church a couple of times. Once he got his license, our "dates" consisted of him coming over on Saturday or Sunday afternoons and hanging around with our friends. And would you believe he actually had a "Wolf Whistle" on his car?

Since I was still fourteen years old, I just took it for granted that I wasn't allowed to go out on a Saturday night date, even though some of the girls from my class were already dating. Then one Saturday morning I got a call from a girl I knew at school, and she wanted to introduce me to her cousin. She had hoped that he and I would go out that night with her and her boyfriend on a double date. As it turned out, his name was Bill, and he was the "new boy" in school all the girls were talking about. Without even thinking it over, I said yes. Now all I had to do was get the okay from Mom and Dad. When I told Mom I had a date that night, she said I'd better ask Dad first. Of course, when I told Dad I had a date that night, he asked, "who said you could go?" But before I could think of anything to say, he just laughed and said it was okay.

As far as I was concerned, the date was a disaster. We went to a drive-in movie in Adrian, and since this was my first real date, I was so shy I didn't know what to say or do. When I got home at 1:00 a.m. from the date, Mom was waiting up, and she wasn't happy. They forgot to tell me what time I had to be home!! Needless to say, he didn't ask me out on another date - at least, not right away! My other friend and I saw each other for a while longer, and then broke up later in the summer when he went up north to stay with friends.

Meanwhile, Pat had graduated from high school and got a job at a grocery store in Toledo, and also started dating her future husband, Earl. He had recently been discharged from the Marines after being stationed in Korea, where he had won a Silver Star. He had also gone to high school in Petersburg before enlisting in the service.

In August, I saw into Bill again and he asked me out on another date. After we'd dated for a while, he asked me to go steady. When I had met Bill's family I learned his Grandpa had died recently in an accident. His grandparents had a farm on Morocco Road, a couple of miles south of town, so Bill's parents had decided to move from Dundee to Petersburg to help his Grandma with the farming. Bill helped his Dad on the farm after school and on weekends, as well as setting pins at the bowling alley in Deerfield.

He and I double dated with some of his classmates and their girlfriends, as well as some friends of his, Berta and Larry, former neighbors from the Dundee area. I remember what an Elvis Presley fan I was, and when "Love Me Tender" was released, I could hardly wait to see it when it came to the theater. Our dates usually consisted of going to a drive-in theater in Adrian or

Toledo and to a restaurant afterward. One of our favorite places to eat was a drive-thru restaurant in Holland, Ohio, that served hamburgers the size of a dinner plate! The hamburger and an order of fries was more than enough for two people. We also went to a place in Adrian called Bummies for burgers after a Saturday night date. Bill was an excellent skater (better than me!), so we occasionally went to the London Skating Rink, and in the fall would go on hayrides with friends from school.

Back then, the price of gas was less than 20 cents a gallon, and saddle shoes and bobby sox were "in," as were poodle skirts and jeans with "pegged" (tight-fitting) legs. When Elvis Presley made his first appearance on television, like the rest of the girls my age, I wouldn't have missed it for the world. Two of my favorite shows on television were "I Remember Mama" and "Ozzie and Harriet". One day I read in a movie magazine that Ricky Nelson liked his hamburgers with just lettuce, cheese and mayonnaise. Of course, I had to try it, and that's still my favorite hamburger today.

When Bill got his class ring, he gave it to me to wear on my left hand. The ring was way too big, so I did what all the other girls did who were going steady. I put layer after layer of thin adhesive strips around the ring until it fit me. Then many coats of my favorite fingernail polish until it was smooth. It took a while, but it looked quite nice when it was finished. One thing about having a boyfriend who had a car - I didn't have to walk to school anymore! He picked me up every morning for school and dropped me off at home afterward, and we'd sometimes go to my house for lunch. The following spring, Bill and I went to the High School Prom (he was a junior) and I got to wear my first formal dress, as well as getting my first corsage. We had a great time and Mom and Dad actually let me stay out past my 12:00 curfew.

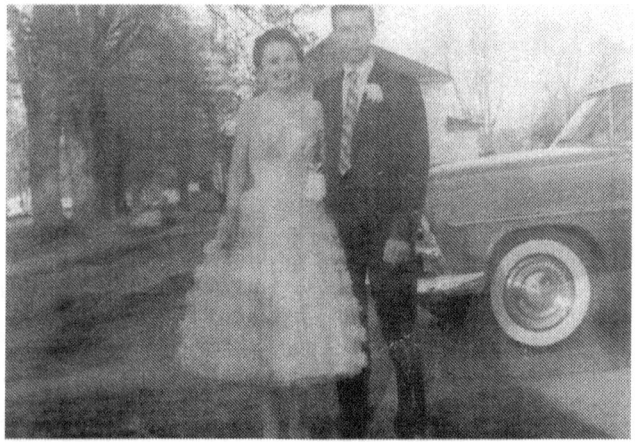

Kay and Bill…Prom Night!!!

In July of 1955, Pat and Earl got married and I was a bridesmaid in their wedding. Pat was a beautiful bride and everyone had a great time at the reception afterward at a place outside of Petersburg called "The Barn." They lived in Dundee when they were first married, then moved to an apartment in Petersburg.

When we went back to school in the fall, it was Bill's Senior year and my Junior year. One of the classes I took was Driver's Ed, and I had to learn on a standard shift car, even though I'd probably never have to drive one again. When I finished the class, I passed my test with flying colors, but with Dad using his car to go to work, I rarely drove, unless I drove Bill's car.

About a month before school started that September, I got a job at the telephone office in Petersburg, working as a part-time operator after school and on weekends. Aunt Edna worked there during the day and I continued to work there until shortly before I graduated from school.

Bill was working for my Uncle Louis at his gas station and helping his dad on the farm. The following spring when he graduated from school, his Mom and Dad gave him a new 1956 Chevrolet (a Bel Air, I believe) for his graduation gift. It was light blue and white, complete with fender skirts. Shortly after graduation, he got a full-time job at a factory in Tecumseh and worked part time at his brother Walt's gas station in Clinton in the evening.

When Bill's Grandma passed away, his parents decided to buy a farm near Clayton, a small town in Lenawee County, almost an hour's drive from Petersburg. Bill's younger brother, Ted, was still in school and attended Onsted high School until graduation. Bill still managed to find time between jobs and dating me to help his Dad on his new farm.

Shortly after I started school in the fall of 1956, Bill gave me an engagement ring for my seventeenth birthday while we were at the drive-in theater (how romantic). He asked me to grab his jacket off the back seat, and said he had something he wanted to show me. Then he took out the ring and proposed. I have to admit, I knew he'd been looking at rings and was kind of expecting an engagement ring for my birthday. We decided to get married two weeks after my graduation, on his Mom and Dad's wedding anniversary, June 14. When I went back to school the following Monday, my teacher had heard about my engagement and asked me to come to the front of the class and show them my ring. How embarrassing – was my face red!!

I knew my Senior year would be busy, what with my job at the telephone office, school and making plans for a wedding, but I continued working at the telephone office until a couple of weeks before the wedding. Once I was engaged and planning a wedding, Mom and Dad relaxed the rules a little and I'd spend the night once in a while at Bill's parents. I slept on the living room sofa, and Bill's Dad liked to tease me and say they had me sleep in the living room so they could keep an eye on me. So, while my classmates were in New York and Washington D.C. on their Senior trip, I was addressing wedding announcements and shopping for my wedding dress. I graduated the last week in May and Mom and Dad had a party for me afterward.

Bill and I had bought a small one bedroom mobile home and he and his Dad moved it to their farm a couple of weeks before the wedding. It was fairly new and already furnished except for a television, which Bill's Mom and Dad gave to us for a wedding gift.

A MARRIED WOMAN!

Bill and I were married on June 14, 1957. He was nineteen and I was seventeen when we married, and although I would have preferred a big wedding like Pat and Earl, Bill wanted a small wedding. So small, in fact, that he only wanted our parents, best man and maid of honor (Larry and Berta) to attend. My sister, Pat, and Aunt Ellen both decided nothing was going to keep them from my wedding, so I didn't find out until later that they hid in the church balcony at St. Peter's and watched the service. After the wedding, Bill and I, along with our parents and attendants, went to a restaurant in Adrian called the Rock Inn and had dinner, complete with a wedding cake. Mom and Dad gave us money as a wedding gift, and the next day while Bill helped his Dad with the farming his Mom and Grandma VanVleet (she was visiting from California) and I went shopping for groceries and some of the things I needed to set up housekeeping. Since I didn't know much about preparing a meal, Bill's mom was a big help and as it turned out the best mother-in-law a girl could hope for. I still use some of the recipes she gave me. About a month after Bill and I got married, Bill's Mom had a family reunion at their farm, and much to our surprise, many of the relatives that came brought wedding gifts for us.

We'd only been married a couple of months when Bill got laid off from the factory, and shortly after that, Dad helped him get a job at the dairy in Toledo where he worked. Soon after that, we decided to move closer to Toledo and moved our mobile home to a trailer park in Lambertville, Michigan. With the added expenses after the move, I got a job over the holidays at a store in a nearby mall. The extra money really helped with the bills and Christmas, but after the holidays I got laid off and had to start job hunting again. Since I already had experience as a telephone operator, I got a job with the Whiteford Telephone Company. This was larger than the telephone company I had worked at while going to school, and covered several communities in the area. With both of us working full time, we decided to buy a small piece of land near Petersburg and build a house. We bought a wooded acre south of town and on the same road as Bill's sister and brother-in-law, Shirley and Del. With help from our families, we got the land cleared enough to move our mobile home onto it and started our plans to build.

Our plans changed when we learned I was pregnant and also that the telephone company I worked at was planning on switching over to a dial system, which meant there would no longer be a need for telephone operators.

Since we knew we'd need more room when the baby arrived, we sold our mobile home and moved briefly to an apartment in Lambertville, then to another apartment above the telephone office in Petersburg. By this time, they were also preparing to switch over to a dial system. Since I was almost eight months pregnant and found the steps to the apartment difficult to climb, and we had also acquired our first dog, Butch, we went house hunting. We found a cute little two-bedroom house on Madison Street in Petersburg and rented it for $50.00 a month. It was perfect! It was so close to Mom and Dad's, I could walk over to see them whenever I wanted. Pat and Earl lived on the other side of town, so I had my sister nearby, too. My brother, John, had graduated from school in June of 1959 and was planning on enlisting in the Navy.

About this time, we still had money from the sale of our mobile home, so Bill decided to take over a franchise on a Marathon gas station in town. He worked midnights at the dairy and then days at the gas station, burning the candle at both ends. To make matters worse, he kept investing more money into the business, had to hire someone to work part time for him while he got a little sleep, and over-extended credit to some of his customers. We soon found ourselves in such a financial bind that I couldn't even afford to buy baby clothes.

One evening early in September, Mom invited me to a "ladies aid meeting" at her house. Because I wasn't a member of the ladies aid I was a little reluctant about going, but Mom insisted and I gave in and said I'd be there.   Pat had taken me to my Doctor's appointment in Toledo that afternoon, and we'd stopped on the way home so I could buy a little undershirt for the baby. I was so thrilled with my purchase, I decided to take it with me to Mom's and show it to her. When I got there, she called me into the living room. Imagine my surprise when I walked into the room, baby shirt in hand, and there were all my former co-workers from the telephone office. They'd brought refreshments, as well as a bassinette full of gifts for my baby. They'd all parked their cars down the street, and I never suspected a thing. I'd thought on my last day of work I'd probably never see any of them again, so it was great seeing them and catching up on what they'd all been doing since we'd last seen each other.

WE BEGIN OUR OWN FAMILY

Not long after that, I woke up one morning when Bill came home from work (he was still working midnights), and I went into labor. The first person I called was my doctor, then Mom and Dad and Pat. Pat came over and helped me get ready for my trip to the hospital. Our daughter, Patricia Marie, was born on October 2, 1959 at 6:00 p.m. She weighed 8 pounds, 6 ounces and was absolutely perfect. As soon as Bill called Mom and Dad, they were on their way to see their first grandchild.

Due to her polio, it was too difficult for Mom to hold her new granddaughter, but Dad more than made up for it. They came over to see Patti almost every day, and when I took her to Church, Dad would hold her through most of the service. If she fussed or needed a bottle, he'd take her back to the church vestibule and look after her. One morning, while talking to me on the phone, he heard Patti crying in the background. Within minutes after he'd hung up the phone, he was there with a rocking chair, picked her up and rocked her to sleep.

Soon after Patti was born, Bill got laid off at the dairy, and also had to close the gas station. We rented a house in Sylvania, Ohio, and Bill went to work for an insurance company in Toledo. It was right around this time that we found out I was pregnant again. When the insurance job didn't pan out, Bill got a job with a car dealer in Blissfield, Michigan. So we moved again, this time to a big old farmhouse outside of Riga, Michigan. Bill worked on a commission basis for the car dealer, and since the country was in a recession, there were some weeks we didn't have any money coming in at all. Whenever we had money, the first things we bought were baby food and milk, and as the time drew near for our second baby, I weaned Patti from the bottle. During this time we had our own "great depression," and we no longer had our own car, so Bill drove one of the "demos" from the car dealership.

As the weather started to turn colder, and we couldn't afford coal for the furnace, we burned just about anything we could find outside to keep warm. We fell behind on the rent, and when the electricity and telephone were shut off, we finally turned to Bill's parents for help. Well, my father-in-law got in touch with my Dad and he came over as soon as he could get there. Bill's Dad ordered a load of coal for the furnace, and Dad took me to the grocery store and told me to buy whatever I needed, and he'd pay for it. And between the two of them, they got the electricity and telephone turned back on. As for the back rent we owed, Bill's Dad told him he could take some corn out of his corn crib to sell, and use the money for the rent. They were both definitely life savers that day.

THE 1960'S: OUR FAMILY GROWS

We went to Bill's Mom and Dad's for Thanksgiving, and two days later on November 26, 1960, our son Robert Louis was born. He weighed six pounds and eleven ounces, and named after one of Bill's friends. He also had Bill's middle name, Louis. Bill's Mom stayed with us for a few days to help, just as she'd done when Patti was born. She said, "Since Bobby is so little, I'll take care of the cooking, cleaning and whatever else that needs to be done. You take care of the baby!" When she came over, she'd brought fruit and vegetables she'd canned, as well as meat from their freezer. She went back home after a few days and I really hated to see her leave.

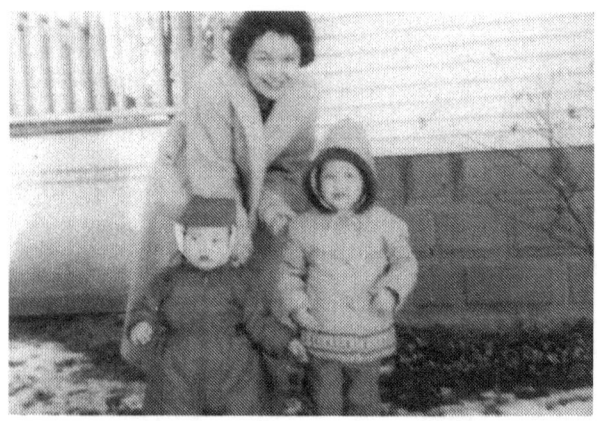

Kay, Bob, and Patti

By this time, John had enlisted in the Navy, went to Great Lakes Naval Station, and then on to the Navy's Electrician's school. He had also gotten married around this time. After a couple years of schooling, he was stationed on the U.S.S. Grampus, a diesel-powered submarine, and then later aboard a nuclear submarine, the U.S.S. Swordfish. Later, he was stationed in Hawaii, and while there, he and his wife had two children, a girl and a boy. Mom eventually bought a typewriter so she could write letters to John and his family.

Bill and I were still struggling financially, so in June, 1961 we took the kids with us and went to Ann Arbor to look for work at University of Michigan Hospital. It was quite a drive from where we lived, but we were desperate to find work. So while Bill stayed in the car with the kids I went inside, filled out an application and had an interview. There was an opening in Radiology for an X-

Ray Aide, so they sent me to Radiology for an interview and to observe what all the job entailed. As it turned out, it was assisting the doctors with both upper and lower "G.I.'s." When I was offered the job, I accepted. At that point, I would have taken any job they had offered me. After taking care of the necessary paperwork at Human Resources, I went back out to the car and told Bill I got a job. He and the kids had been waiting a couple of hours, and even sat in the car through a thunderstorm. So then it was his turn to go inside while I waited in the car. When he returned to the car, he had a job working in Messenger Service. We were both working for slightly above minimum wage, but it was a start.

After we started working, we looked for a place to rent closer to Ann Arbor, and found a four-bedroom house in a subdivision in Milan that we rented with an option to buy. The upstairs needed finishing and when we decided we could do the work ourselves, Bill's Mom and Dad loaned us the money for the down payment. In less than a year, we'd both moved on to different jobs at the hospital and increased our income a little more. I got a job as a Correspondence Clerk in the business office, and he was working as an Ambulance Attendant in the Emergency Entrance. Bill eventually went to school and had on-the-job training to become a Respiratory Therapist.

We eventually finished the upstairs in our house, built a garage and added a family room. We each had our own car now and Bill took on a part time job working for the vending machine company that serviced the hospital, ARA. When Bill was offered a full time position with ARA, he quit his job with the hospital.

In November of 1963, my Grandma Redick passed away while Bill was up north deer hunting. Bill's Mom offered to keep Patti and Bobby at her house while I spent some time with Mom and went to the funeral. Later that month, I was at work at the hospital when I heard President Kennedy had been assassinated. Everyone at work was in shock and like the rest of the country, we were glued to the television for the next several days. Patti was only four years old at the time, but still remembers watching the funeral procession on television, and the cadence of the drums.

My brother, Jim, graduated from high school in 1964, and went to work part time in Ann Arbor while going to Cleary College for a year, and then he worked the following year at Bendix Aerospace in Ann Arbor.

I found out in the summer of 1965 we were expecting our third child, with a due date in January, 1966.

In late January, my Grandpa Redick passed away following several years of heart problems. Then, on February 2, 1966, I went into labor at 4:00 p.m. and our second son, William Louis, Jr. was born at 8:00 p.m., and weighed eight pounds and fifteen ounces! He was a good "little" baby, who had a good disposition, and how that boy loved to eat!

My Grandpa Gaertner passed away later that month, when he became ill after walking up town to Uncle Glen's IGA grocery store. It was an extremely cold day and when he walked inside the store, he became faint. When he refused to go see his doctor, my cousin, Louie took him home to rest while he went to get his wife to stay with him for a while. When he returned with Fran just a few minutes later, Grandpa had passed away peacefully, still lying in the same position as when Louie had left him. He was 89 years old.

In March of 1966, Jim was drafted into the Army, and after he was finished with his basic and AIT training, he was stationed at an Army helicopter base on the edge of Tan Son Nhut Air Base near Saigon, Vietnam. Bill's younger brother, Ted, had graduated from school, gotten married and was living near Flint when he too was drafted into the Army. He was also stationed in Vietnam.

When Billy was about a year old we decided to sell our house in Milan and buy a farm. After we started looking, we found a 40-acre farm on a gravel road just west of Tipton, Michigan. The house was small (two bedrooms), and needed a lot of work, including a furnace. We moved into the house on our tenth anniversary and the first thing Bill did was start buying the equipment he needed to farm the land. Even though I was raised in town and knew absolutely nothing about farming, Bill taught me how to drive a tractor so I could help him, and when he was done planting his crops he started working on the house. While working on the living room addition, Bill got some help from our fathers, his brother-in-law, Del, and my brother, John, who'd been discharged from the Navy.

Since living in the country was a new experience for the kids, they were curious about just about everything new to them. One evening while Bill and I were installing the new cupboards in the kitchen, Bobby came in to tell us about a black and white cat that was in the back yard. Bill's reply? "Go catch it; it'll make a nice pet." Well, it wasn't long and we heard him crying. And we smelled him coming before we saw him come into the house. The "cat" was actually a skunk that had sprayed him just as he bent down to pick it up. He undressed in the basement and I gave him a bath and washed his clothes. At the time, he also wore glasses, so we wound up taking his glasses to the Ophthalmology clinic at the hospital, where they dismantled them and put them through a special cleaning solution.

Also, after we'd moved to the farm, Bobby started a bug collection. Each time he caught a bug he'd put it in a jar or bottle, poke holes in the lid and put it in a box on the back porch. His collection was so big, you could hear all the "angry buzzing" whenever you stepped onto the porch. He eventually traded his bug collection to a friend of his for a wild gold finch in a cage.

One day Bill decided to buy the kids a pony that our neighbor had for sale. That little "stallion" named Billie didn't want <u>anyone</u> on his back, and would buck off anyone who tried. He got loose a couple of times, and after Bill had to chase him down, he decided maybe having a pony wasn't such a good idea after all. In fact, I can still picture him in his Bermuda shorts and flip-flops chasing the pony through the soy bean field.

While living on the farm, we had a male black Labrador retriever we'd gotten from Pat's husband Earl. He was a good hunter, and all Bill had to do was get out his gun and Blackie was raring to go. He was also really good with the kids, but bad news for any cat that came onto our property. He did, however, tolerate a barn cat named Frances that we had. Later on, we got another dog, a little black poodle that the kids named Sammy.

By now I was working as a Registrar in Outpatient Registration at University Hospital. As a matter of fact, I was working there when they first started bringing patients in by helicopter. The landing pad was right outside the clinic where I worked, so we all crowded around a window in one of the exam rooms to watch it land.

It was around this time that the family got word that Bill's brother, Ted, had been wounded in Vietnam. We were told that he had stepped on a land mine and had suffered traumatic amputation of both legs. When he arrived back in the United States he was taken to an Army hospital in Colorado, and we immediately made arrangements at work so we could drive out to see him. Coincidentally, his wife had given birth to their first child, a boy, the same day he'd stepped on the land mine. They stayed on in Denver where his wife taught school and they also had another son.

When the vending company Bill worked for in Ann Arbor got a contract with a factory in Tecumseh, he was given a management position and was now working closer to home. And after putting in a few applications, I got a job in the business office of a local hospital as a Service Representative

THE 1970'S: YEARS OF CHANGE...AND NEW CHALLENGES

At around this time, Dad's employer, Sealtest Dairy, was closing its Toledo facility where he worked. He was given the option of retiring or moving to the new facility near Cleveland. Dad was not too thrilled with either option, but was more inclined to retirement after spending his entire life in southern Michigan.

In January, 1972, Pat, Earl and their kids came over to have dinner with us and watch the Super Bowl. Pat and Earl now had three children, Brian, who was almost 11 years old, Cyndi, who was 9 and Kristina, who was 7. They had bought a home in Petersburg and Earl was a dispatcher for a trucking company. Little did we know when they left that day that Earl would die in a car accident between Deerfield and Petersburg the following month.

Needless to say, Pat was absolutely devastated and having a pretty rough time, and with Dad choosing the early retirement option from the dairy, it allowed him to be there for her and the kids. Later on, he and Mom bought a travel trailer and took Pat and the kids on a much needed vacation to some theme parks in Florida.

Not long after that, Bill decided we needed a bigger farm. So we sold our farm and bought an 80-acre farm south of Onsted, Michigan, where the kids already attended school. In addition to farming, we raised pigs and cattle to take to market. It was nice having a home that didn't need remodeling or some sort of repair, and the back yard had many dwarf fruit trees - apple, pear, peach and cherry. It also had a big yard between the barn and road where the kids liked to play ball with their friends. There was also a ditch that ran across the property behind the barn where they liked to play tug of war with their friends, and a loft in the barn where they could play basketball.

By now, Bill had quit his job with the vending company and started working at a factory in Adrian. We lived close enough to his folks that he and his Dad helped each other with their farming. We had several couples in the neighborhood we'd get together with for cookouts and playing cards. We even bought a couple of snowmobiles and would go riding with some of our friends on trails through the fields and woods in the winter. In fact, one of the couples we were friends with, Babe and Virgil, would one day be my daughter's in-laws.

Due to our mounting debts on the farm, I looked for another job and found a secretarial position at a factory in Addison, where I worked for Research & Design and also proofread for the Sales and Advertising Department.

Later on, after Patti married Babe and Virgil's son, Doug, they had a son, Douglas Jr. Babe and I were best friends and loved to go to garage sales, play cards or just get together for coffee and talk about our grandson. However, late in the fall of 1975, Babe developed a persistent cough and when she finally went to the doctor, she learned she had lung cancer, and passed away less than six months later.

In February of 1976, my brother Jim, moved to Arizona, and attended Arizona State University in Tempe. He graduated from ASU with a Bachelors Degree in Journalism in 1979, and began working for The Arizona Bank as a procedures analyst.

Bill and I had our share of disagreements over the years, but one evening in June, 1976, we got into a heated argument after I came home from work. I wound up leaving that evening and we divorced in May, 1977. Bill remarried soon after the divorce, sold the farm and moved to Florida a few years later.

I also remarried several months later, however, it was soon apparent the marriage wasn't going to work. And although I had custody of Bob and Billy after Bill and I divorced, I soon let them go to live with their dad due to the stressful situation in our home. He and I separated several times over the next few years, attended counseling, but eventually divorced.

THE 1980'S: THE KIDS START THEIR OWN FAMILIES

In May, 1980, Bob got married and he and his wife, Jackie moved to Clinton, Michigan where Bob worked at a feed mill. The following year in April, they had a son, James Robert.

While Billy was living in Florida, I missed him terribly, and whenever his Dad came to Michigan to see his family, he brought him over to see me. We also wrote to each other and I even managed to go down to Florida a couple of times and spend a little time with him.

Patti and Doug had two more children, Deanna was born in May, 1980 and Steven was born in January, 1982. Bob and Jackie had another son, Jason, born in May, 1984. Later on, Billy had moved back to Michigan after he turned 18, and he became the proud father of a son, David John, born in August, 1988 . He was named after my brother, John, who had passed away quite sudden at work on September 15, 1987.

Pat had called me at work to tell me our brother, John, had passed away at work that morning with an aneurysm. The entire family was in shock. Dad and Jim had an especially difficult time dealing with his loss, and after the funeral Dad would go out to the cemetery every day. John was only 46 years old, and he enjoyed life so much, especially going to NASCAR races and taking "racing" vacations in Arizona to see Jim. In fact, he had already made reservations to fly out to see Jim in October to attend a race. Pat and I flew out to Arizona two months after John had passed away and the three of us spent Thanksgiving together.

THE 1990'S TO THE PRESENT

The following year while Dad and Mom were vacationing in Florida, Dad was hospitalized after he had passed out one morning. He was admitted to a local hospital and told he needed to get a pacemaker before he returned home. When he returned to Michigan, he contacted a cardiologist at St. Joseph's hospital in Ypsilanti for follow-up care. He seemed to be doing alright until December 17, 1989, when he was hospitalized again, this time at Flower Hospital in Toledo. He was diagnosed with septicemia and admitted to Intensive Care, but his condition gradually worsened. Jim came home from Arizona to spend some time with him, and Dad passed away at 79 years of age on January 3, 1990. Ironically, Dad's sister, Meta, and his best friend and fishing "buddy" Fritz, had both passed away with cancer just days before Dad.

Later, there was an especially touching moment at the funeral home when a young man who had known Dad all his life walked in. He lived outside of town and passed by Mom and Dad's house every day. He said if Dad was outside when he drove by, Dad would always give him a little salute. Then he took a couple of steps back and said, "So long, Les", and saluted Dad before leaving. At the funeral service the following day, Pastor Thomas described Dad as a "fine Christian gentleman who loved his family". That pretty much described exactly the sort of person Dad was. He always gave of himself and expected nothing in return.

I had moved to an apartment in Dundee and shortly after that, applied for work at a nearby hospital, in Tecumseh, Michigan, where I worked for the Business Office in Registration and also Switchboard. I went to Church with Mom and Pat at Prince of Peace Lutheran Church in Ida and spent weekends with Mom, Pat and my family.

In May of 1995 I saw my ex husband, Bill one weekend at my daughter's house. He was divorced now, living back in Michigan and working for a trucking company. It was a rather cool day and he gave me his jacket to put on while he and I sat on the tailgate of his pickup truck, and he fished in their pond. I saw him again about a month later when Mom and I stopped by to see his house he was remodeling in Onsted. Less than a week later I got a call one evening that he had died in a tragic work-related accident. His untimely death was a terrible shock for our children and the rest of his family, and extremely difficult for them to deal with. But, I'll be forever thankful that he and I had that time together near the end to just visit and talk about our children and grandchildren and spend some time together as a family.

In the spring of 1997 I met someone through a coworker at the hospital. His name was Leo and he worked at a factory in Tecumseh, and had been divorced for quite a few years. Everyone in my family liked him and in a way, he kind of reminded me of Dad. He was six months older than me and we seemed to like the same things and have a lot in common. After dating for six months, we were married at the Courthouse in Toledo on Halloween, 1997. We were living in Tecumseh when we both retired in 2001, and moved to Adrian shortly after that.

Pat had moved in with Mom when Mom's health had started deteriorating. Her osteoarthritis had gotten worse and she sometimes needed help getting dressed. She also had macular degeneration and was considered legally blind, which resulted in frequent injuries due to falls. I tried to get over to see her every day, and she, Pat, Aunt Edna and I would often get together and play dominos in the morning, or just visit over a cup of coffee.

Jim moved back to Michigan for two years in 1998. He was married in April of 2000 in Ida, Michigan, to Shirley Morris, whom he had worked with while working for the State of Arizona in the early 1990's, and had kept in touch with while in Michigan. Following their wedding, Jim moved back to Arizona. He and Shirley presently reside in Phoenix, and he works for FedEx Freight. Shirley still works for the State of Arizona's Department of Environmental Quality.

Jim and Shirley came to Michigan for a visit in early September, 2003, and shortly after they returned to Arizona, Mom lost her balance one evening, fell in her kitchen and injured her back. After a short time in the emergency room and Xrays, Mom was sent home with some pain medication. When she didn't improve over the next few days and started hallucinating, I went to stay at her house to help Pat take care of her. A few days later, Mom was admitted to a hospital in Saline for five days then discharged to a nursing home in Tecumseh, and after a few days she was transferred to a nursing home in Adrian.

Pat and I saw her every day at lunch time and I'd usually go back in the evening to make sure she ate her dinner, since she could no longer feed herself. She was admitted to the hospital on November 15, after it was determined she'd had a heart attack and had also developed pneumonia. We notified Jim and Shirley, and then Pat and I stayed by her side around the clock. Between the pain and the morphine, Mom was not herself during her final days. She passed away on November 19, 2003, at 8:00 in the evening at the age of 89. Pat, my oldest son, Bob, and I were with her.

Three months later, Leo and I separated after it appeared as though we had "jumped the gun" when we decided to get married. We divorced amicably and still remain friends today.

Later, while Pat and I were preparing to sell Mom's house, Pat found out she had some heart blockages that required catheterization and stents. The following year, she was diagnosed with breast cancer and underwent radiation therapy after having the tumor removed. She'll be taking medications and going to her doctors for regular checkups until she gets a "clean bill of health" again. This past January, she slipped on some ice outside her home one Sunday morning when leaving for Church. The fall resulted in two fractures in her leg that required surgery and hospitalization, as well as months of recovery.

Pat, Jim, and I try to get together at least once a year. Usually, Jim and Shirley come to Michigan in the late summer or early fall for a week. In September, 2006, Pat and I flew to Las Vegas and were met there by Jim and Shirley. Not only was this my first time in Las Vegas, Jim and Shirley also took me to several attractions I'd never seen, including the Grand Canyon (on my birthday) and the Hoover Dam. Incidentally, the area we went to view the Grand Canyon was the Hualapai Indian Reservation, where the new Skywalk was recently constructed. I even had my first In-n-Out hamburger!

Our family is planning a reunion in August for the decendents of John and Anna Gaertner. Its been quite a while since we've gotten together with our cousins and their families, and we're hoping for good weather and a large "turnout".

We're also looking forward to Jim and Shirley's visit in September. The four of us are planning on spending a couple of days together in northern Michigan while they're here, as well as other side trips and points of interest. Jim is planning our itinerary and making our reservations. Perhaps if all goes well, Pat and I will fly out to Arizona next year.

I'm also looking forward to my Summerfield High School Class of 1957's 50th reunion. This will be in October and I can hardly wait to see my former classmates, many of whom I've not seen since graduation. I'm sure, we've all got a lot of catching up to do.

Although I'm semi-retired now, I still work part time as a Switchboard Operator at the hospital, where I've been employed for the past 16 years. It seems I've come full circle…starting out my working career at a switchboard and now working at one again.

My family is also growing by leaps and bounds! I have a great grand son, Ethan, four great grand daughters,

Shelby and Emma (Mom would be so happy!) Skylar and Mara.

And although I'm no longer looking for old buttons and lace, I still enjoy going to antique shops. Last summer, I took my son, Bob, and my sister Pat to an antique shop in Brooklyn, Michigan, where we browsed through so many of the things that remind me of those early years of my life, and it makes me realize all over again what a good childhood we had. Pat and I try to get together at least once a week, and at some point during our visit, one of us will usually say, "Do you remember when …" Once again the years melt away as we relive some nearly-forgotten joy from those days when we were kids and realize, despite the setbacks along the way, how fortunate we really were to have been born into such a loving, happy family. It turns out that hindsight really can be such a blessing.

ABOUT THE AUTHOR

"Hindsight" is Kay Tabbert's first book. It's a vivid personal recollection of growing up in a small, rural southeastern Michigan town in the 1940's and 50's, filled with many of the types of warm memories that so beautifully fill in the pages of our lives, and taking place in a simpler time so very different from the frenzied America of the early 21st century. She lives in Adrian, Michigan, near the same region in which she grew up and in which much of her story takes place.

www.ingramcontent.com/pod-product-compliance
Lightning Source LLC
Chambersburg PA
CBHW031256280526
45784CB00004B/1871